12 IMPORTANCE OF THE POWER OF SEX IN A RELATIONSHIP.

Exploring a grip of intimacy

By

Dr TIMOTHY KESSINGTON.

approval from the publisher or creator.

TABLE OF CONTENT

ABOUT THE AUTHOR

Dr. TIMOTHY KESSINGTON is a licensed psychologist in the state of texas. he is a certified counselor on marriage and relationship/mental health. He is passionate to the core to see people in relationships happy and couples achieve the best out of every relationship

Introduction:

A romantic relationship cannot exist without sexual intimacy. It enables people to connect on a deeper level, resulting in a sense of emotional closeness and bonding. Sex has undeniable power in a relationship, and it can influence many aspects of a couple's dynamic. Understanding the role of sex in a relationship can help couples navigate challenges and maintain a healthy, fulfilling partnership, which has been widely researched and explored. In this essay, we will investigate the power of sex in a relationship by looking at how it affects various aspects of a couple's dynamic.

CHAPTER 1

The Importance of Sexual Compatibility.

The degree to which two people's sexual desires, needs, and preferences align is referred to as sexual compatibility. A healthy relationship requires sexual compatibility, as a lack of compatibility can lead to frustration, dissatisfaction, and conflict. A variety of factors can contribute to sexual incompatibility, including differences in libido, sexual preferences, and sexual experiences. As a result, open communication about sexual needs and desires is critical for couples to ensure they are on the same page.

CHAPTER 2

Communication's Role in Sexual Intimacy.

Communication is an important aspect of sexual intimacy in a relationship. Open and honest communication can make it easier for couples to express their sexual desires and boundaries, resulting in a more fulfilling sexual experience. Misunderstandings, unmet needs, and feelings of dissatisfaction can all result from a lack of communication. Couples must establish healthy communication patterns to improve their sexual connection.

CHAPTER 3

The Effects of Sex on Emotional Intimacy.

Sexual intimacy in a relationship can help to strengthen emotional intimacy. During sexual activity, the release of oxytocin can promote bonding, trust, and feelings of closeness. A lack of sexual intimacy, on the other hand, can lead to feelings of disconnection, resentment, and emotional distance.

Prioritizing sexual intimacy in a relationship can thus assist couples in maintaining emotional closeness.

Chapter 4:

The Relationship Between Sexuality and Physical Health.

Sexual activity can be beneficial to one's physical health. Regular sexual activity has been linked to better immune function, less stress, and lower blood pressure. Sexual activity can also be used as a form of exercise, promoting physical fitness and cardiovascular health. As a result, incorporating sexual intimacy into a relationship can benefit physical well-being.

CHAPTER 5

The Relationship Between Sex and Mental Health.

Sexual activity can also be beneficial to one's mental health. Endorphins released during sexual activity can increase feelings of pleasure while decreasing stress and anxiety. Furthermore, sexual intimacy can increase self-esteem and feelings of self-worth, contributing to overall mental health. A lack of sexual intimacy, on the other hand, can lead to feelings of depression, anxiety, and low self-esteem. As a result, prioritizing sexual intimacy in a relationship can improve mental health.

CHAPTER 6

The effects of sexual trauma on sexual intimacy.

Sexual trauma can have a significant impact on a relationship's sexual intimacy. Individuals who have experienced sexual trauma may struggle with feelings of shame, guilt, and anxiety in the presence of sexually active partners. Sexual intimacy should be approached with sensitivity and understanding, with open communication and respect for each other's boundaries being prioritized.

Chapter 7:

The Influence of Age on Sexual Interaction.

Age can influence sexual intimacy in a relationship. Hormonal changes can cause changes in libido and sexual function as people age. Physical health issues and medications can also have an impact on sexual uncouples must prioritize open communication and be willing to adapt to changes in sexual function as they age.

Chapter 8:

The Effects of Stress on Sexual Intimacy.

(The Effects of Stress on Sexual Intimacy in a Relationship). Stress can cause a decrease in libido and sexual desire. Furthermore, stress can cause tension and anxiety, making it more difficult to connect sexually with a partner. To maintain a healthy sexual connection, couples should prioritize stress management techniques such as mindfulness, exercise, and therapy.

Chapter 9:

The Impact of Culture and Society on Sexual Intimacy.

Sexual intimacy in a relationship can be influenced by culture and societal norms. Different cultures have different attitudes toward sex among students, which can influence how people approach sexual intimacy. Furthermore, societal norms and expectations can exert pressure and influence sexual behavior. To improve their sexual connection, couples must understand and respect each other's cultural backgrounds and values.

CHAPTER 10

The role of sexual experimentation in a relationship.

Sexual experimentation in a relationship can be a healthy

and fulfilling part of it.
Experimenting with new things
and exploring each other's
sexual desires and boundaries
can strengthen the sexual
connection and promote the
need for couples to approach
sexual experimentation with
respect, open communication,
and a willingness to prioritize
each other's comfort and
boundaries.

Chapter 11:

The Effects of Adultery on Sexual Intimacy.

Infidelity can have a devastating effect on a relationship's sexual intimacy. Betrayal and breach of trust can cause feelings of resentment, anger, and emotional distance, making it difficult to connect with sexual couples who need to prioritize open communication, set boundaries, and work through

any underlying issues to
rebuild trust and intimacy.

Chapter 12

Sexual Relationship Maintenance Techniques.

Maintaining a healthy sexual relationship necessitates effort and communication. Prioritizing time for intimacy, practicing open communication about sexual needs and desires, and experimenting with new sexual experiences can all help to improve a relationship's sexual connection. Prioritizing

physical and emotional health
through exercise, stress
management, and therapy can
also have a positive impact on
sexual intimacy.

Conclusion:

Sexual intimacy is an important aspect of any romantic relationship. It can improve emotional and physical intimacy, promote mental and physical health, and strengthen partner bonds. However, various factors such as communication, culture, trauma, and age can all have an impact on sexual intimacy. To maintain a healthy sexual connection, couples must prioritize open communication, respect each other's boundaries, and adapt to changes in sexual function and desire. Understanding the power of sex requires a couple to prioritize hinges and cultivate a fulfilling relationship.

www.ingramcontent.com/pod-product-compliance
Lightning Source LLC
Chambersburg PA
CBHW050755250726
48662CB00005B/2227